It's Not About Dying-It's About Living

Making Difficult Decisions In The Name of Love

Michelle Crowell, BSN, RN

It's Not About Dying-It's About Living

Making Difficult Decisions In The Name of Love

Michelle Crowell, BSN, RN

I devote this book to my precious parents Bobby & Charlotte Crowell and my dear grandmother Lois Johnson and all the thousands of patients I have had the privilege to care for in my 24 years of nursing. You are loved and missed.

Introduction

Over the last twenty four years that I have spent in the nursing field, fifteen of which have been hospice, I have had to deal with many difficult conversations that revolved around end of life. So many people struggle to talk about death and the things that happen surrounding dying. Some might even say having discussions about death while one is yet alive is taboo.

I believe however that it is very necessary and vital. Too many times I have experienced the heart breaking decisions that families must make about their loved one's care. Confusion, uncertainty, guilt, love, anger and many other emotions are often displayed. When information about one's medical condition is not properly explained, this often leads to unrealistic expectations of treatment and life expectancy. Many times decisions for aggressive treatments are made that may not have otherwise been chosen if the knowledge had been presented up front and before life and death hung in the balances.

I, myself, have experienced what it is like to love someone and have to make difficult choices at the end of life. My father was diagnosed with kidney cancer and told there was nothing left to do for him. Although, I was a newer hospice nurse, I was still a daughter who was broken, devastated and longed to find a "fix" for my daddy's disease. I allowed my dad to be in a hospital for a total of eighteen days on two separate occasions while he was sick. During those times, my dad experienced some procedures that not only did not relieve his pain or extend his life, but caused him more pain, more self-awareness about his condition and ultimately caused more suffering. I'm so thankful his pain ended just ninety two days after diagnosis, but I would do anything to go back and not allow him to have been prodded on just so I could keep him longer.

My intentions on writing this book are to shed light to exactly what happens in most people at the end of life, to explain that letting go of aggressive treatment is not giving up hope, and to bring comfort for those who will one day have to face making difficult decisions for those that they love.

It's not about dying...it's about living...

In today's world of modern medicine, there are so many medications, treatments and interventions that help to expand one's life span for many years. Often, cancers, heart disease, respiratory problems, diabetes and other diseases can be healed or stabilized. But what happens when they cannot? When the disease has progressed to a point of no return and the treatments are no longer working, what do you do? Have you made an advance directive? Have you discussed with your family whether or not that you want life sustaining treatments? Do you know the difference between aggressive and palliative or comfort care? Does CPR bring everyone back to life? These are some questions that I hope I will be able to answer and help you make an informed decision about your life or someone that you love's life.

Aggressive Care versus Comfort Care:

Aggressive care describes a particular approach to a life-threatening illness or condition. A patient receiving aggressive care will attempt every medical treatment in order to prolong life. Chemotherapy, dialysis, radiation therapy, surgery, antibiotics, CPR, and other medical interventions designed to preserve and prolong life would be considered aggressive care.

Comfort care describes care that is focused on relieving symptoms and optimizing comfort. When a patient can no longer benefit from active treatment, comfort care can allow them a better quality of life at the end of life. This care focuses on not trying to cure the disease but to alleviate the symptoms that diminish quality of life.

So many times, we do not understand the meaning of what these treatments may or may not do. At times, all of the treatments listed above may be very appropriate. My objective is to explain how some of these treatments may not be the best choices in end of life care and how they affect the body in a negative way.

We will look at the following treatments:

- CPR
- Feeding tubes
- IV fluids and TPN
- Dialysis
- Pain management

CPR

CPR is the abbreviation for cardiopulmonary resuscitation. It is used when sudden death occurs that is unexpected. The key word in this definition is the word unexpected. A motor vehicle accident, a heart attack in a forty year old male, lightening striking an individual are examples of death that is unexpected. CPR in this case is very appropriate and can often save a life. CPR was never meant to be performed on patients who are at the end of life and are facing a terminal illness. Statistics show that less than 1% of terminally ill patients survive CPR. So why is CPR done on these people at end of life? One of the main reasons this occurs is due to lack of knowledge.

Everyone should have an advance directive in place. What do I mean by an advance directive? Merriam-Webster defines advance directives as "a legal document (such as a living will) signed by a competent person to provide guidance for medical and health-care decisions (such as the termination of life support or organ donation) in the event the person becomes incompetent to make such decisions."

Most people do not even think about a living will. Statistics show only about 29% of individuals even have one. Why is this so? Fear? Thinking they won't need one? As the daughter of a man who was fifty eight years old and working every day when he was diagnosed with cancer, let me tell you that I wished my father had completed one earlier in his life. But to him it was unnecessary because he was going to live a long time and it was "foolish" to think about it that early.

When people hear the words DNR or Do Not Resuscitate, it implies that something will not be done for them. I've had so many people tell me "yes I want everything done for me." Or "yes do what you can for momma." But when I explain the concept of what DNR means, there is often a change of opinion. If I were to ask you this question how would you respond? If you have already died, do you want me to break your breastbone into, puncture your lungs etc. to bring you back into your body? 9 out of 10 people will say "No, if I'm already gone, let me go on in peace." I love how some states have adopted the term AND, which stands for Allow Natural Death. This is so much more comforting and lets individuals know that it is natural to die. And that death is actually a part of life. Doing CPR will not bring you back into a healed body but if your medical team is able to bring your heart beat back, then you will be intubated and placed on a ventilator. Then the decision becomes harder for your family as to when to take you off life support. Would you still want to have CPR knowing all of this? It does not mean that your caregivers will not do everything they can for you while you are alive, it just means that once you have died that you do not wish to be attempted to be brought back into a fragile, sickly shell that you once knew as your body.

In end of life there is almost always a loss of appetite. Sometimes this loss of appetite can be caused due to constipation, nausea and pain. Oftentimes, once the underlying issue is resolved then so will the appetite issue.

In cases where there is not a reversible cause then many patients and caregivers may look for artificial means of nutrition such as feeding tubes and IV nutrition.

Feeding Tubes

Feeding tubes are usually used when a patient is no longer able to swallow or has a condition that prevents them from orally taking in their nutrition. There are several kinds of feeding tubes.

NGT are nasogastric tubes and are placed through the nostril down past the esophagus into the stomach. PEG-Percutaneous endoscopic gastrostomy & G-tubes-gastrostomy tubes are placed surgically into the stomach through the abdomen. Feeding tubes also serve a great purpose for individuals who have had an unexpected accident, injury or illness that they may ultimately recover from. However, in patients who are facing end of life illnesses the feeding tubes may not be in the best interest of the patients.

I am from the South so I understand all too well about the importance of eating. We eat at special occasions, we eat to celebrate, and we eat when we are happy, sad, and mad. We bring food to families when there is an illness or death at their home. So I understand just how hard it is to face when someone we love is unable to eat. We don't want the thought that "mamma" is going to starve to death or "daddy" is going to die if he doesn't eat. This isn't the case at all and we will discuss this further as we go along.

The bad news about feeding tube in end of life situations is that there are many issues that may occur. These are just a few:

- Possible aspiration issue with any feeding tube but especially with NGT
- Diarrhea often caused from feedings which may lead to break down in skin integrity in a bed bound patient resulting in a wound.
- Discomfort at insertion site of a PEG/Gtube.
- Possible infection at times at insertion site.
- At end of life feedings can keep patient more alert to surroundings and symptoms of dying process
- Extra fluid may cause congestion or fluid overload

It may be easier to make the decision not to have a feeding tube placed when our loved one or even we can no longer swallow versus removing the feeding tube.

TPN/IV Fluids

TPN, otherwise known as Total Parenteral Nutrition is the procedure in which all nutrition is provided intravenously and the normal way of eating and digested is bypassed completely. TPN is delivered through a central venous line that is usually placed in the neck or armpit area. TPN has all essential vitamins and minerals necessary to maintain weight and produce energy. TPN is replacing the normal way of eating by giving all of the nutrition through an IV line.

Why is it not good to give TPN at the end of life? Here are a few reasons:

Complications/Side effect of TPN:

- Infection at the site
- Pneumothorax from insertion of CVL-this means collapsing of the lung when the IV is placed into the main vein of the body.
- Thrombosis-this means blood clot in the body.
- Cardiac arrhythmias- this means that the heart is not in a normal rhythm.

- Electrolyte imbalances- the body is made up of different electrolytes such as calcium and sodium. Oftentimes, there becomes an imbalance when giving artificial nutrition.
- Fluid overload-this means that the body has received too many fluids and cannot dispose of them correctly.

Many people will want to give their loved ones IV fluids at the end of life. They believe this will help the dehydration and help when they are no longer wanting to eat or drink. Let us look at why we should not give IV fluids and what dehydration and starvation truly mean to a person who is at the end stage of living.

Here are the main reasons for not giving IV fluids at the end of life:

- IV fluids do not alleviate thirst.
- Best form of hydration is good oral hygiene using oral swabs and lubricants.

- Most of end of life patients will not experience overwhelming thirst and usually ice chips or sips will satisfy this.
- IVF often cause fluid overload- the body cannot process the extra fluid and overwork the kidneys, edema, CHF. This causes extra fluid to go out into the tissues causing more swelling, fluid in the lungs, more pain, and increase in sensitivity of the body's senses.

Dehydration

Dehydration is the absence of an appropriate amount of water in the body. When there is not enough water in the body then the body is not able to carry out its normal functions.

Dehydration is a normal part of the dying process. Many caregivers will become fearful of this process and desire to have IVF/TPN or other aggressive measures. It is very important to understand the process to help alleviate any fear that harm is taking place.

When dehydration occurs at the end of life, endorphins are produced. This is the body's natural "morphine" so to speak. This causes euphoria, a natural state of happiness or well-being, to occur. The only negative effect usually may be dry mouth, in which one can use mouth swabs to moisten lips/inside of the mouth.

When we use IVF/TPN we prevent dehydration and the patient is very aware of any pain or discomfort and we do not let nature take its course.

In most areas food is a sign of comfort, love and family. Therefore, when a patient is no longer eating, families often feel like the patient is going to starve when in reality that is not the truth.

As the activities of the body change so is the amount of energy or nutrients that are needed. If a patient is bed bound then they will not need the amount of calories that they did when they were up moving around. The body is brilliant and recognizes this.

As the need lessens for food the body will reroute it's metabolism to slow it down, thus requiring less intake. This continues to happen as the body continues to decline and so will the metabolism and nutrient level.

What this means is that a patient will not starve like in the case of a normal healthy individual. This is part of the body's way of slowly shutting down the body one system at a time and the patient will usually not be hungry or experience any discomfort from not eating. This process is often more painful for the loved ones to watch and they often have a harder time dealing with this. Many people can live 2-3 weeks without food but usually only 8-10 days without water. This process of the body slowly shutting itself down is the natural circle of life and nothing to fear.

Dialysis

Dialysis is when a patient's kidneys have failed to the point that they are no longer able to filter the body's waste anymore naturally. A central venous line access will be placed in the body to deliver dialysis. I like Merriam-Webster's definition of dialysis- "the process of removing blood from an artery (as of a kidney patient), purifying it by dialysis, adding vital substances, and returning it to a vein." Patients can be on dialysis for years and years but as time moves forward and other body organs become diseased or begin to fail, one may choose to stop dialysis.

The decision to end dialysis is often a hard one but is usually decided when the quality of life a patient has is no longer good. The patient is often bedbound and suffering from multiple issues. It is one of the hardest choices to make and the goals of comfort only are often the reason for the decision.

Pain Medication at End of Life

There is no evidence that opioids such as morphine hasten the dying process when patients receives the right dose to control the symptoms that they may be experiencing. In fact, research states that using opioids to treat pain or shortness of breath near the end of life may help a person live a bit longer. Pain and shortness of breath can often be exhausting. Patients near the end of life have limited strength and energy. Treating these symptoms oftentimes slow down the rate of decline, if only for a few hours. There is no need to fear medications to treat symptoms. Education can be provided for by your caregivers such as hospice, palliative care, and hospital or by whomever you have chosen to have your care provided for.

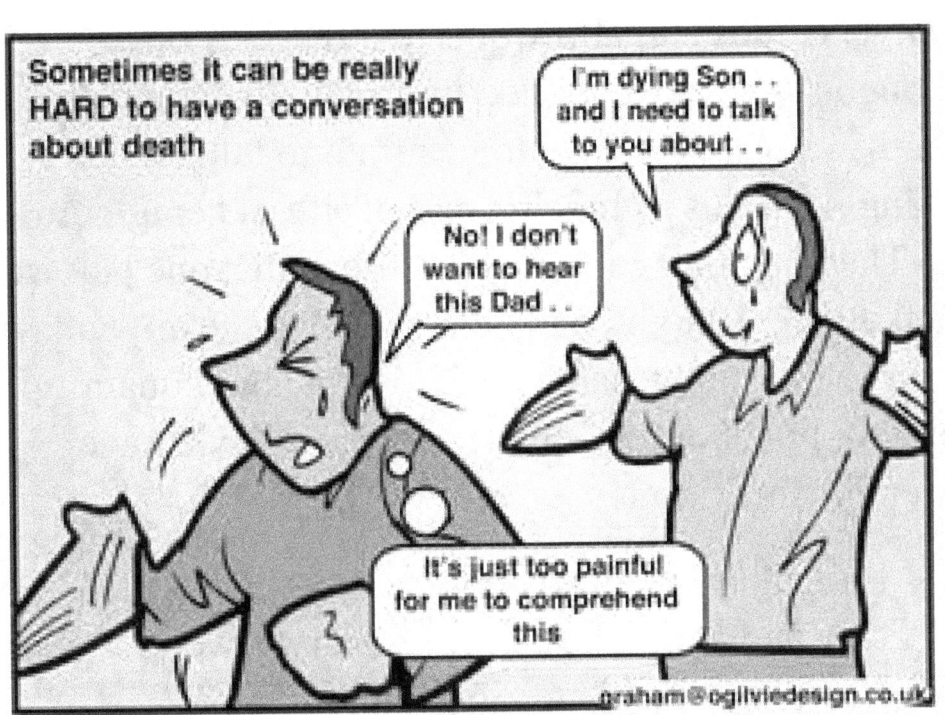

It is important that we as individuals encourage these hard conversations. Sometimes even for your physicians and others it may be hard to have these "talks" as it causes us to look at our own mortality. But it is necessary to help facilitate these conversations and allow open expressions of thoughts, concerns and feelings by both patient and family. You don't have to be afraid to talk about dying. Dying is as much a part of life as being born is. The one thing certain about life is that one day we will all die. But you have the choice to make you last days the best they can be. Life is not about quantity of days but about the quality of the days we have been given.

- Have those talks when loved ones about their care and about the care you want as well.
- Get a living will, advanced directive, power of attorney. You are never too young
- Let your choices be known up front about what your wishes are.
- Mostly, learn to make every day count and live to the fullest.

Life is a journey and each one of our journeys are different. Don't be afraid to ask questions of your caregivers, doctors or any other medical profession. Don't be afraid to talk to your loved ones. You don't have to be afraid to die because it's not about dying but it's about living…

Michelle Crowell has been in the nursing field since 1993. She has spent the last fifteen years in hospice which is her passion. It is her goal to spread the knowledge about end of life care and to help dispel the myths surrounding hospice care. Her desire is that all persons receive the level of care that they may need to be adequately cared for with the best quality available.

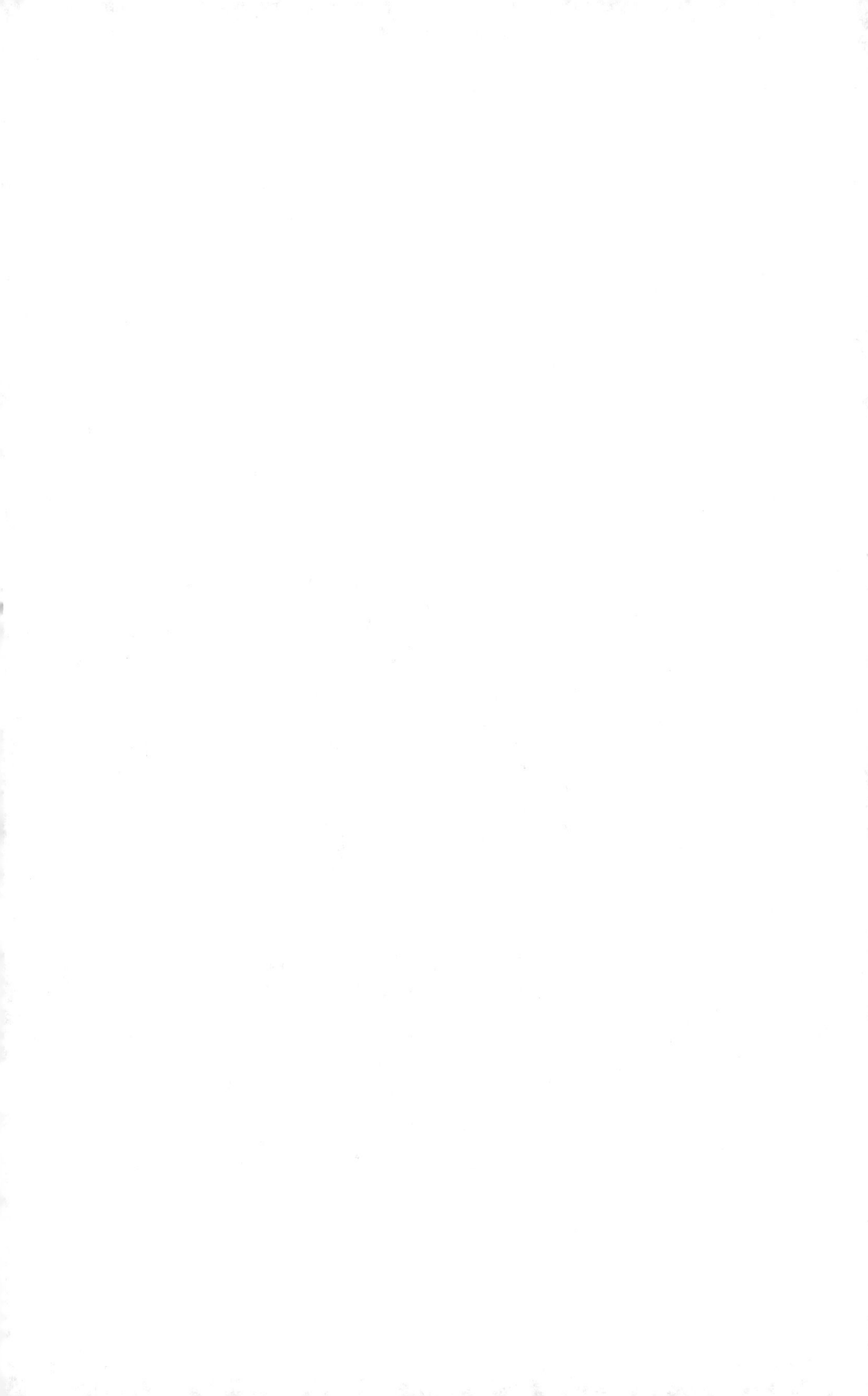